Overview

Stomach ulcer is a physical affection, which appears on the lining of the stomach. It may appear in other parts of the digestive system (e.g. duodenal ulcers). For any type of ulcer, the term used is stomach ulcer. However, detailed explanations are given in the sections of this text. The most prevailing symptom is the sensation of burning in the center of the abdomen. This is not the only symptom, and some other people might face indigestion and heartburn. It is important for the person to see a doctor if there is suspicion of suffering from stomach ulcer. The most aggravating symptoms that urgently require seeing a doctor/specialist are (1) vomiting blood and (2) sudden and sharp pain in the stomach, which firmly worsens.

The particular cause of the stomach ulcer is the break within the layer that protects the stomach lining. Therefore, the stomach acid hurts the stomach lining, determining the pain. It was believed that stomach ulcer appeared as a cause of stress or because eating some particular aliments, but in fact it is the result of an infection with Helicobacter pylori (H. pylori) bacteria or of an overuse of non-steroidal anti-inflammatory drugs (NSAIDs).

There are not exact researches counting the exact numbers of people suffering from stomach ulcer, as it is a common affection. However, some studies came up with the result that at least 1 in 10 people is susceptible of having a stomach ulcer in their lifetime. Most commonly it appears at people over 60 years.

The good news is that stomach ulcer can and will be healed, with proper treatment, in less than 60 days. The treatment depends on the initial causes and almost all the times are medication, in adapted dosage. In some cases, complications of stomach ulcer can appear, but they are rather uncommon. It is important to know these complications can be extremely serious and life-threatening. They include bleeding at the site of the ulcer, the perforation of the stomach, or a gastric obstruction.

What is stomach ulcer?

The dictionary definition of ulcer shows it is *a local defect, or excavation of the surface of an organ or tissue, produced by sloughing of necrotic inflammatory tissue.*

What is commonly known as *stomach ulcer* is medically known as *peptic ulcer*. The differences in terms are explained below. Particularly, it is a *loss of tissues lining the lower esophagus, stomach, or duodenum.* The Farlex Partner Medical Dictionary defines it as *an ulcer of the upper digestive tract, usually in the stomach or duodenum, where the mucous membrane is exposed to gastric secretions.* The Medical Dictionary of The American Heritage defines *peptic ulcer* as *a sharply circumscribed loss of the mucous membrane of the stomach, duodenum, or any other part of the gastrointestinal system exposed to gastric juices containing acid and pepsin.* Pepsin is an enzyme released by the cells in the stomach and that degrades food proteins into peptides.

This type of ulcer can be either acute or chronic. The acute ones are usually multiple and only on the surface. They do not show the usual symptoms of a stomach ulcer, and heal without leaving scars. The most damaging ones are the chronic ulcers, as they are deep, persistent and symptomatic, and the muscular coat of the stomach cannot regenerate. After it is treated, there is a scar left, and the mucosa of the stomach heals completely.

The factors which cause stomach ulcer include: excessive secretion of gastric acid, inadequate protection of the mucous membrane, stress, heredity, and the use of certain drugs. Recent research shows that the ulcer is caused by the bacterium *Helicobacter pylori.*

It is important to know that stomach ulcer is neither cancerous, nor contagious. Some types of ulcer (e.g. duodenal ulcer) can sometimes become malignant. Its size usually ranges between an eighth of an inch and three quarters of an inch.

In some cases, stomach ulcer is a symptom of other condition or disease. For example, it appears in the case of *mastocytosis* (= a condition characterized by infiltration of mast cells into the tissues of the body. Mast cells are connective tissue cells which release chemicals including histamine that are very irritating and determine itching, swelling, and fluid leakage from cells.) Also, if a person bleeds from stomach ulcer, it develops further iron deficiency anemia. Stomach ulcer appears not only in case of adults, but children also suffer from it.

Different types of ulcers

Commonly, people refer to stomach ulcer, but there are many others examples, less known. The term *stomach ulcer* is a broad affection, and it includes several types of ulcer. There are in fact seven different types of ulcers that can affect the digestive system. The ulcers are named especially after the location within the body. However, the peptic ulcer can be traced anywhere in esophagus, stomach or duodenum.

The most common types of ulcer are: (1) peptic ulcer; (2) gastric ulcer; (3) duodenal ulcer. The peptic ulcers are the ones caused by pepsin, and are normally found in the stomach or duodenum. Pepsin is also present together with hydrochloric acid, in the stomach lining. If the peptic ulcer is detected in the stomach, it is called gastric ulcer. Its symptoms are more specific. If the peptic ulcer is present in the duodenum, it is named a duodenal ulcer. It develops in the first part of the small intestine.

Research shows that duodenal ulcers are the most common in the Western World. Lucile Packard Children's Hospital at Stanford documents showed in 2013, that in the United States of America, around 25 million people have gastric and duodenal ulcers at least once in their lifetime. Also, more than 40 thousands Americans have surgery because of issues or symptoms connected to ulcer, each year, and around 6 thousand of Americans die every year, because of stomach ulcer related complications.

Other types of ulcer are the following:

(1) esophageal ulcer occurs in the lower end of the esophagus, and are generally associated with a case of acid reflux. It is also known as GERD (Gastro Esophageal Reflux Disease);

(2) bleeding ulcer originates in a peptic ulcer that has been left untreated. It is referred to as a bleeding ulcer. It is the most dangerous type of ulcer, as it the same with an internal bleeding. It is recommended to see a doctor immediately if a person shows specific symptoms;

(3) refractory ulcer is in fact peptic ulcer that has not healed after three months of treatment;

(4) stress ulcer is actually a series of lesions/lacerations, located in the esophagus, stomach or duodenum. Normally it manifests at patients who are critically ill or severely stressed.

What causes stomach ulcer?

Helicobacter pylori – H. pylori

It was believed that stress and spicy foods are the main causes of stomach ulcer. More recent research has come to a different conclusion. The results show that stomach ulcer is caused by a bacterium known as *Helicobacter pylori* – H. pylori. It is not known how it spreads, but some say it can be taken through close contact, such as kissing, or even through food and water. The infection with this bacterium is pretty usual, and the infection does not produce immediate symptoms. The bacteria live mainly in the stomach lining and can be taken by people of all ages. It irritates the stomach lining and increases the stomach's vulnerability to damage from the stomach acid. Still, it is not exactly known how some persons are more vulnerable to H.pylori effects than others.

Acid and Pepsin

Other causes for ulcer formation are gastric acid and pepsin. In some stomach ulcer cases, there is an increased amount of hyperacidity of the gastric juice. Some theories state that both gastric and duodenal ulcers occur in families. The statistics say that relatives of persons with gastric ulcers have three times the expected number of gastric ulcers. The number is the same in the case of duodenal ulcers.

The hydrochloric acid and pepsin – an enzyme which digests proteins - destroy the intestinal or gastric lining of a person's stomach, which manifests into a stomach ulcer.

The stomach prevents the damage from pepsin and hydrochloric acid by creating a mucus coating, which acts as a shield for the stomach, produces bicarbonate and assures the circulation of blood to the stomach lining in order to assist in both cell renewal and repair. If any of these actions is perturbed, there are conditions for an ulcer to appear.

Use of NSAIDs

NSAID is the short for non-steroidal anti-inflammatory drugs that are prescribed to treat a wide range of conditions, such as pain, inflammation (redness and swelling) or fever. The most well-known NSAIDs are aspirin and ibuprofen. The list of short-term conditions for which NSAIDs are used as treatment includes: headaches, painful periods, toothache, soft tissue injuries (sprains and strains), and infections such as the common cold. The same type of medication is used for treating long-term (chronic) conditions such as: most types of arthritis, including rheumatoid arthritis, other forms of inflammatory arthritis and osteoarthritis, chronic back pain, and chronic neck pain.

A person who uses NSAIDs must be attentive with the increase in the risk of experiencing a heart attack, stroke, or heart failure. The risks highly depend on the dosage, the period of time they are used, and the type of drug which is used. However, every person who suffers from any heart disease should not take NSAIDS unless there is no other alternative or medication that can bring the same benefit. The high-risk groups for NSAIDs uses include the persons with a history of heart issues (heart attack, stroke or heart failure), people aged over 75 or over, smokers, people with diabetes, and people with high blood pressure. Moreover, NSAIDs are not recommended normally to persons who are in one of the following situations: are pregnant or breastfeeding, have a history of significant kidney disease, have a history of significant liver disease, have active stomach ulcers or are at high risk of developing stomach ulcers.

When using NSAIDs it is necessary to consider the possible side effects. They are unlikely to appear on short term use, but it is not the case when used on long-term basis. The main side effect appears within the gastrointestinal system, respectively indigestion, allergic reactions and *stomach ulcer*. When prescribed to older patients (aged over 55), people who have had previous stomach ulcers or people who need long-term NSAID treatment, medication to suppress stomach acid is also prescribed.

The usual NSAIDs prescribed in Europe are:

(1) diclofenac

(2) ibuprofen

(3) naproxen

(4) celecoxib

(5) mefenamic acid

(6) etoricoxib

(7) indomethacin

(8) aspirin (in doses greater than 600mg)

Lifestyle factors

The development of stomach ulcer may also be determined by psychosomatic factors. When a person faces a long period of physiologic stress, they risk developing stress ulcer. From a pathological and clinical point of view, it differs from a chronic peptic ulcer, as it is more acute and highly likely to produce hemorrhage. Also, the condition of stress ulcer is generally put together with severe trauma, surgery, advanced malignancy, extensive burns, and brain injury.

Alcohol, smoking and spicy foods may also favor the appearance of stomach ulcer, even if it is no prove about it. However, these are conditions that worsen the symptoms of stomach ulcer. For example, smoking may make the treatment less effective.

The risks of developing an ulcer can include, besides what was explained above, the following:

1. Chronic disorders such as liver disease, emphysema, rheumatoid arthritis

2. Improper diet, irregular or skipped meals

3. Excess alcohol consumption

4. Zollinger-Ellison syndrome

5. Family history of ulcers

6. Type of blood

Stomach ulcer symptoms/signs

The symptoms of stomach ulcer vary, and do not show in the same way in everyone. However, as soon as possible the signs described below appear, or at least a part of them, the person suffering should see a doctor for diagnosis and treatment. The most common symptoms of stomach ulcer are the following:

1. Vomiting

Usually, it begins with nausea, making difficult for the person to complete daily task and have a normal live. In short time, the nausea becomes sickness and ends with vomiting throughout the day. Without treatment, the symptom could rapidly result in in serious dehydration and illness, as well as malnutrition, as a result of the food not being digested properly by the body.

2. Blood in the vomit

Together with the previous symptoms, one may notice blood in the vomit. When traces of blood are found, it is a sign the ulcer has advanced and is highly damaging the interior of the stomach. In other words, the internal bleeding seeps into the stomach.

3. Abdominal pain

As the ulcer burns the wall of the stomach, the patient might experience pain in the abdomen area. The pain is noticeable most of the time, but it increases in intensity after eating a meal, or as the eaten food passes from the stomach into the intestines. The extreme pain will come in episodes, but will gradually worsen.

Taking antacids (indigestion medication) may relieve the pain temporarily, but it will keep coming back if the ulcer is not treated.

The bacterium H. pylori can also cause painful inflammation of the stomach and small intestine lining. Pain can also be caused by a buildup of gases and constipation.

4. Darker stools

The internal bleeding seeps into all the digestive system. This also occurs as a result of tissue dying and being absorbed through the stomach and into the gut. As a consequence, the stools are darker, and sometimes might contain traces of dark-colored blood. The more blood is noticed, the larger is the risk and the ulcer damage.

5. Rapid weight loss

As it affects the appetite, the stomach ulcer can determine huge and quick weight loss. The ulcer usually stops the person suffering from eating as much as they usually do, given the pain they feel. The weight loss will also occur as a result of vomiting, which is a common occurrence for people who have ulcers.

6. Hunger pains

Usually, after a large meal, someone might feel all of a sudden something very similar to hunger pains. Even if it feels identical with it, it is not the same. In fact, the body is digesting the food, and the pain is caused by digestive fluids and juices increasing in the stomach, and sometimes even leaking through the stomach walls.

7. Bloating

This symptom appear on a regular basis around the abdomen area, making people unable to wear tight clothes and making them feel like they have gained weight. Actually they did not. For it to be a symptom of stomach ulcer, it should be associated with other signs.

8. General gassy feeling

Normally it is a result of an ulcer causing intestinal obstructions, allowing gas to build up as the food is broken down. It feels like a result of gas building up in the stomach and working up through your body.

9. Bad Breath

H pylori organisms present in stomach acid create ammonia, which results in bad breath.

10. Heartburn

Even if this symptom usually appears from different other reasons than stomach ulcer, it is common for this affection as well. It is also called acid reflux, or GERD. When acid is low, digestion of food becomes slow and difficult. The result is that food sits in the stomach too long and gives off gases which can cause burning sensations in the stomach and throat.

11. Constipation / Diarrhea

When H. pylori causes low stomach acid, food is not processed properly causing undigested food to be released into the intestine. The diarrhea may only happen infrequently, or it may happen almost daily, depending on how chronic the infection is.

12. Dehydration and malnutrition/Anemia

The regular vomiting and the discomfort when eating determine serious dehydration and malnutrition. This occurs as the body expels nutrients that have not been properly digested yet, as well as fluids consumed during the day.
Anemia or iron deficiency is closely linked with an H. pylori infection. When an H. pylori infection has caused low stomach acid, it becomes particularly difficult to digest protein (which contains iron).

Together with the ones listed above, someone should consider as symptoms of stomach ulcer the following: the sensation of burning in the stomach, cramping, gnawing, and aching that comes in waves that last for several minutes. The pain is usually diminished in the morning, when the secretion of gastric acid is lower and after meals when the food is present in the stomach. The pain increases in intensity before meals and at bedtime. Sometimes the symptoms appear within a few days in a week, and reappear weeks or months later.

A stomach ulcer affects the nerves which surround it. The nerves that are affected become agitated, causing the person pain. Stomach ulcers may cause hemorrhages due to erosion of a major blood vessel, or a tear in the wall or the person's intestine or stomach. The result may be peritonitis or an obstruction of the person's gastrointestinal tract due to either swelling or a spasm in the area of the person's ulcer.

Other secondary symptoms appear, as a result of the first ones. The list includes:

1. Anxiety

2. Depression

3. Fatigue or Low Energy

4. Headaches or Migraines

5. Skin Problems

6. Pre Menstrual Stress

7. Sinus Problems

8. Sleep Problems

Did you know that?

... some types of stomach ulcers are not painful and are noticed only when a complication develops, such as bleeding from it.

...   it is always recommended for a person facing the symptoms of stomach ulcer to have the diagnosis confirmed by a health professional.

... even if it might be detected only when the ulcer bleeds, 90% of all types of ulcer are easily curable.

... unattended ulcers can start bleeding - and this is potentially the most dangerous condition of all

Diagnosis

A correct diagnosis of the stomach ulcer is the key for a proper treatment and healing process. It is highly recommended that a health professional sees the person with the symptoms of an ulcer, and firstly test it for the infection of the H. pylori bacteria.

There are several ways to diagnose the ulcer.

Endoscopy/gastroscopy and Biopsy

Endoscopy is an accurate form of diagnosis for ulcers. An endoscope is a long, flexible tube with an attached camera. It is threaded down your throat and esophagus into the stomach and duodenum. Using the camera, the doctor views the digestive tract and stomach cavity and sees if there are any ulcers present. During the procedure, the patient might be given a mild sedative injection and have the throat sprayed with a local anesthetic to make it more comfortable to pass the endoscope. An endoscopy/gastroscopy is usually carried out as an outpatient procedure, which means the person does not have to spend the night in hospital.

A small sample (biopsy) is taken from the lining of the stomach and small intestine during an endoscopy. While the diagnosis is very accurate for ulcers, the results from the tests performed on a biopsy are not always consistent.

X-rays/the barium test

The x-ray shows an outline of the esophagus, stomach and duodenum. Before taking the X-ray picture, the doctor asks the patient to swallow a white liquid, called barium or barium meal. This forms a coating on the digestive tract and makes an ulcer more visible on the X-ray. X-ray can only detect some ulcers, but not all. X-rays cannot detect the presence of any H. pylori bacteria. Double contrast films are sometimes done to clearly define the mucosal pattern in the upper gastrointestinal tract.

Breath test

It is a non-invasive test, but also extremely expensive. It involves using a radioactive carbon atom to detect H. pylori bacteria. The first breath is captured and sealed in a small plastic bag. After that, the patient has to drink a small glass of liquid containing radioactive carbon as part of a substance (urea) that will be broken down by H. pylori. Thirty minutes later, a second breath sample is captured. If the second breath sample contain the radioactive carbon in the form of carbon dioxide, this indicates an infection with H. pylori.

Blood tests

A blood test checks for the presence of H. pylori antibodies, not for the bacteria itself.

Stool antigen test (HPSA)

This is a very accurate test check, which sees if the substances that trigger the immune system to fight an H. pylori infection (H. pylori antigens) are present in your feces (stool). It is the only known test that shows an accurate result regarding the presence of H. pylori status in a person's body. ELISA HPSA test is the most advanced and accurate test available, and is the recognized benchmark test used in this field. It is the only test that provides conclusive proof of the presence of H. pylori bacteria.

Stomach ulcer treatment

The purpose of the medical treatment for stomach ulcers has four phases: (1) to relief the symptoms; (2) to enhance the process of healing; (3) to prevent any further complication; (4) to prevent the reappearance of other episodes. The treatment, however, differs from patient to patients, as it depends on individual needs and responses. The treatment usually includes the medication, the patient care, and the patient education. The medication is based on different types of antacids (e.g. cimetidine). For example, antacids as magnesium hydroxide and aluminum hydroxide ease the pain caused by ulcer, by lowering the level of gastric hydrochloric acid and pepsin in the stomach.

There are a number of types of medicines, to include H2-blockers, mucosal protective agents, and proton-pump inhibitors. To treat H. Pylori, these medications are used in conjunction with antibiotics. Should medications prove ineffective, or should complications arise, surgery may become needed.

H2 receptor antagonists are a class of drugs that block the action of histamine on parietal cells (specifically the histamine H2 receptors) in the stomach. This decreases the production of acid. Examples of H2-blockers include Ranitidine, Cimetidine, Nizatidine, and Famotidine. The person usually takes a single dose at bedtime in order to start healing a duodenal ulcer over a four week period of time, and a gastric ulcer in six to eight weeks. Side effects are uncommon, but may include diarrhea, headaches, dizziness, rashes, and tiredness.

Proton-pump inhibitors (PPIs) are a group of drugs whose main action is a pronounced and long-lasting reduction of gastric acid production. They are the most potent inhibitors of acid secretion available. They modify the production of acid in the person's stomach by stopping their stomach's acid pump. An example of a proton-pump inhibitor is Omeprazole, which has ten-times the ability to suppress stomach acid than an H2-blocker, healing a duodenal ulcer in two to four weeks. The side effects of these are usually mild, but can include headaches, diarrhea or constipation, feeling sick, abdominal (tummy) pain, dizziness, rashes.

Mucosal protective agents protect a person's stomach's mucous lining from acid. Examples of this type of medication include Misoprostol, and Sucralfate. Non-prescription forms of these medications include antacids and bismuth subsalicylate.

Antibiotics can be administered to persons who are infected with the H. Pylori bacteria, causing ulcers. Examples of antibiotics that are commonly prescribed include Tetracycline and Metronidazole, although a doctor may substitute amoxicillin or clarithromycin. The side effects of antibiotics are usually mild and can include feeling and being sick, diarrhea, a metallic taste in the mouth.

In some cases, if the ulcers was caused by NSAIDs, the health care specialist may recommend the change of it. The doctor should advise the use of an alternative painkiller, not associated with stomach ulcer (e.g. paracetamol). It is very important to keep in mind the potential risks associated with continued NSAID use. In this case, the patient is most likely to develop another stomach ulcer and could experience a serious complication, such as internal bleeding.

Together with the medication, dietary modification is recommended and relieving the source of psychological stress. **Very important:** None of the medication referred to in this text should be taken without the prescription from a health professional.

In some cases, for the treatment of ulcer is needed surgery, especially when the patients do not fully cooperate and follow the medical instruction. In other cases, the surgery is necessary if there is scarring of the ulcer, producing obstruction, recurrent bleeding, extreme pain, or perforation. Recent research shows that as time lapses between peptic ulcer perforation and surgery, morbidity and mortality rates increase. Every hour is important.

Gastric ulcers are more likely to require surgery than are duodenal ulcers. The operative procedure most frequently done for a gastric ulcer is subtotal gastrectomy, in which the ulcerous portion of the stomach is removed. This procedure is often done in conjunction with vagotomy, (division of the vagus nerve, which eliminates cerebral stimuli of the stomach muscle and glands, thereby reducing gastric motility and secretion.)

When the doctor takes care of the patient, they need to have information about several aspects of the patient's life. Firstly, the health professional has to assess the family history of stomach ulcer. Secondly, they gather information about the patient's eating habits and how eating affects symptoms. Thirdly, it has to be known whether the patient drinks or smokes and to what extent. Fourthly, the patient shares details about any history of psychological or physical stress such as severe trauma, burns, or other conditions that might produce a stress ulcer. Finally, the doctor needs to know of any drugs the patient might be taking that are irritants to the gastrointestinal tract.

Dietary restrictions are included in all the cases of stomach ulcer, and are limited to those aliments, if any, that an individual identifies with the onset or worsening of symptoms. Exceptions are alcohol and caffeine, both of which are capable of inducing gastritis and promoting erosion of the gastric mucosa. It is generally agreed that what the patient with an ulcer eats is not as important as when it is eaten. Frequent and regular feedings throughout the day, rather than two or three large meals, are encouraged. Patients should not skip meals and should try to have some nonirritating food in the stomach at all times.

At this point, the patient has to change their food habits, and the health professional does a sort of education in this respect. The patient has to follow some of the following rules:

(1) Regulate the types of foods eaten and the manner in which they are eaten. Meals should be unhurried, relaxed, and spaced at regular intervals

(2) Do not eat right before bedtime. Stop eating at least 2 hours before bedtime.

(3) Try to avoid situations of stress and anxiety and develop some effective skills for coping with stress

(4) Drink water at least once every hour when awake. This acts to dilute gastric juices, making them less corrosive

(5) Stop or at least cut down on smoking

(6) Keep alcohol intake to a minimum

(7) Report any side effects of antacids or other drugs to the health care provider. There are alternative drugs if the side effects of one are worrisome

(8) Take prescribed medications exactly as ordered and do not discontinue them without consulting the health care provider

(9) Avoid taking aspirin; develop the habit of reading labels of nonprescription drugs to ascertain whether they contain acetylsalicylic acid. Since some prescription drugs also contain aspirin, inform any health care provider treating a coexisting condition that aspirin cannot be tolerated.

Associated complications

Even if stomach ulcers are not very common, when they appear are extremely serious. The most common is *internal bleeding*, which can be either slow, long term-bleeding, determining anemia, fatigue, breathlessness, pale skin and heart palpitations, or rapid and severe bleeding – causing you to vomit blood or pass stools that are black, sticky and tar-like.

Another complication that might occurs is the *perforation,* when the lining of the stomach splits open. It is a very aggravating situation, as the bacteria living in the stomach might infect the abdomen (peritoneum). The complication is also known as *peritonitis.* In this case the infection can quickly advance into the blood – *sepsis* – and further to other organs. It holds within the risk of multiple organ failure. When left untreated, it can be fatal. The symptom of peritonitis is abrupt abdominal pain, which steadily worsens. Peritonitis is a medical emergency that needs hospitalization. In some cases, surgery is needed.

Gastric outlet obstruction is a complication that manifests when a swollen or scarred stomach ulcer obstructs the usual trajectory of food through the digestive system. The symptoms are: repeated episodes of vomiting, with large amounts of vomit that contain undigested food; a persistent feeling of bloating or fullness; feeling very full after eating less food than usual; unexplained weight loss. The obstruction is confirmed by an endoscopy. In case of inflammation, the medication contains proton pump inhibitors (PPIs) or H2-receptor antagonists to lower the acid levels in the stomach until the swelling disappears. If there is scar tissue, there might be a surgical situation. Sometimes, the treatment involves passing a small balloon through an endoscope and inflating it to widen the site of the obstruction.

Prevention

Even if there is no absolutely sure way of preventing stomach ulcer, a person might follow a series of recommendation to avoid it.

Use NSAIDs in the lowest dose possible. Avoid drinking alcohol when on drugs as of this type.

Protect from infections. It is not known how H. pylori spreads, but there is evidence it can easily be transmitted from one to another through food and water. A high level of hygiene is also recommended (wash the hands frequently, eat foods that have been properly cooked).

Quit smoking, as it aggravates the stomach ulcer symptoms. Moreover, studies showed that smoking while under treatment, slows down the healing process. Also, the patients who smoke have greater chance to develop stomach cancer more than once in their lifetime. Professional healthcare providers should recommend solutions for quitting smoking.

Drink alcohol in moderation. The limit should be of 2 drinks a day for men and 1 drink a day for women. A high level of alcohol consumption is often connected to a great risk for peptic ulcers. Altogether, the use of alcohol in association with NSAIDs causes stomach irritation and creates the background for stomach ulcer to develop. In case of a certain diagnosis of stomach ulcer, the alcohol worsens the symptoms.

Consume less caffeine and acidic foods. Caffeine, acidic foods and drinks (e.g. coffee, orange juice, tomato products) increases the stomach irritation and the risk of getting the H. pylori bacterium. In cases when a person already has ulcer, these products irritate more the lining of the stomach.

It has not been proven so far that spicy foods are a cause of the stomach ulcer. However, these types of meals can worsen the symptoms. They are to be avoided until the ulcer has healed.

Get tested for H.pylori, especially if you are over 60 years old, have history of ulcer or a family history of ulcers. For example, in the United States is estimated that more than 50% of the population older than 60 is infected.

Reduce/avoid stress. If it is not a direct cause, stress surely aggravates it. Acute stress increases pulse rate, blood pressure and anxiety. It is recommended to do relaxation exercise and to apply any other stress reducing strategies. There are several techniques to avoid stress.

- Meditate. A few minutes of practice per day can help ease anxiety.

- Breathe deeply. It usually slows the heart rate and lowers the blood pressure. It is enough to take a 5 minute break and focus only on the breathing.

- Slow down and be present in your life.

- Spend times with friends and family. It is important to speak with others and share experiences, thoughts and so on. It highly relieves the psychological pressure.

- Pay attention to the body, stretch it daily and relax it periodically.

- Decompress. Take short breaks to get away of your problems and just focus to yourself.

- Laugh as much and as often as you can. It is known it lowers cortisol, the body's stress hormone and increases the level of brain chemicals called endorphins that help the mood.

- Listen to the favorite music. It usually lowers blood pressure, heart rate and anxiety.

- Practice a form of exercise. It is not extremely necessary to practice a specific sports, yoga and walking are as good as any. Exercising ease depression and anxiety.

- Find the things in your life to be grateful for. It may be useful to keep a personal journal.

Follow a healthy diet. A specialized diet for ulcer and gastritis puts a limit on the foods that may irritate the stomach. In particular, these are the aliments that grow the level of stomach acid. Spices such as pepper, food such as chocolate, or the aliments high in fat should be avoided. A short list of beverages to be avoided includes:
1. Hot cocoa and cola
2. Whole milk and chocolate milk
3. Peppermint and spearmint tea
4. Regular and decaf coffee
5. Green and black tea, with or without caffeine
6. Drinks that contain alcohol
7. Orange and grapefruit juices

The spices that present a high risk of irritating the stomach are:
1. Black and red pepper
2. Garlic powder
3. Chili powder

Other aliments to be avoided in a healthy diet, for preventing the appearance of stomach ulcer, are:
1. Dairy foods made from whole milk or cream
2. Spicy or strongly flavored cheeses, such as jalapeno or black pepper
3. Highly seasoned, high-fat meats, such as sausage, salami, bacon, ham, and cold cuts
4. Hot chilies and peppers

5. Onions and garlic

6. Tomato products, such as tomato paste, tomato sauce, or tomato juice

It is important to have an equilibrate diet, with aliments from all the food groups. It is recommended to consume fruits, vegetables, whole grains, and fat-free or low-fat dairy foods. Whole grains include whole-wheat breads, cereals, pasta, and brown rice. Also, it is good to choose lean meats, poultry (chicken and turkey), fish, beans, eggs, and nuts. A healthy meal plan is low in unhealthy fats, salt, and added sugar. Healthy fats include olive oil and canola oil.

Stomach ulcer diet

In the case of a predisposition to stomach ulcer, one of the ways to prevent or even heal it is the diet. The main idea is to avoid foods that can irritate the stomach. In this situation, watching the diet requires above all discipline.

Highly spiced and fried foods, long thought to be first causes of ulcer, are now considered to have little effect in the course of an ulcer. However, they do bother some people who already have ulcers. If spicy meals, for example, are always followed by a severe gnawing pain, they should be avoided. It is the same with any other aliment that causes discomfort.

An elimination diet can help determine if any specific food triggers an increase in ulcer symptoms. An elimination diet involves avoiding frequently eaten and common food allergens for two or three weeks, then reintroducing them one by one, and taking note of which ones trigger symptoms.

The real key to keeping gastric juices from attacking the lining of the digestive tract is to keep some food present as much of the time as possible. It is important to eat smaller meals, more frequently.

People with ulcers should eat as many unrefined and high-fiber plant foods as possible. A diet rich in highly processed grains (such as white flour) deprives the body of fiber and protein, which can shield the digestive lining from stomach acid. Some high-fiber foods include spinach, cabbage, broccoli, and Brussel sprouts.

One of the earliest treatments for ulcer flare-ups was milk, which was believed to neutralize stomach acid. However, scientists now know that foods high in calcium increase stomach acid. So while the protein part of the milk may soothe, the calcium may make matters worse.

The question of alcohol's impact on ulcer formation remains unanswered. Many medical experts believe that people who drink heavily are at higher risk of developing ulcers than those who drink lightly or not at all.

Some foods can make ulcers worse, while some provide a preventive and healing effect. Greasy and acidic foods are most likely to irritate the stomach.

To reduce ulcer pain, the following items should be avoided:

1. coffee, including decaf
2. carbonated beverages
3. chilies and hot peppers
4. processed foods
5. salty red meats
6. deep fried foods

Risks of ulcer

In general, women and older people are more susceptible to have stomach ulcers. Recent studies showed that young men are more likely to develop duodenal ulcers, and older women to have gastric ulcers. The explanations lies in the aspirin use.

High dosage of aspiring also develops a risk for stomach ulcer.

Alcohol, tobacco and caffeine highly contribute to the appearance of stomach ulcer. Even if there is no research to prove it, doctors recommend patients to stop taking these elements.

The patients with cancer also present a risk for ulcer, especially when they undergo radiation treatment or chemotherapy. Sometimes, it appears together with some other infections. Previous health problems such as cystic fibrosis, hepatic cirrhosis, Crohn's disease, and HIV also can cause stomach ulcer.

The persons who had it once, are more exposed to having it again.

Natural remedies

Besides medical treatment, there are also a series of remedies which are natural, and some even homemade. In some situations they might heal the ulcer totally, in some other they may ease the symptoms.

Flavonoids - or bioflavonoids (from the Latin word flavus meaning yellow, their color in nature) are a class of plant secondary metabolites.

Flavonoids are compounds that occur naturally in many fruits and vegetables. Foods and drinks rich in flavonoids include:
1. soybeans
2. legumes

3. red grapes
4. kale
5. broccoli
6. apples
7. berries
8. teas (especially green tea)

Some foods and drinks that contain flavonoids — such as citrus fruits and red wines — can irritate a stomach ulcer.

Flavonoids are known as being *gastroprotective,* meaning they protect the lining of the stomach and permit ulcers to heal. There is no side effect of consuming flavonoids in the amount found in a typical diet, but higher amounts of flavonoids may interfere with blood clotting.

Deglycyrrhizinated Licorice

It is plain old licorice with the sweet flavor extracted. One study showed that deglycyrrhizinated licorice might help ulcers heal by inhibiting the growth of H. pylori. Deglycyrrhizinated licorice is available as a supplement.

Probiotics

These are living bacteria and yeast that helps the digestive system to work properly. They are present in many common foods, particularly fermented foods. These include:

1. buttermilk
2. yogurt
3. miso
4. kimchi

Probiotics can be taken in supplement form as well. Studies showed that probiotics are helpful in removing the H.pylori and raise the recovery rate for patients with stomach ulcer.

Honey

Depending on the plant it is made from, honey can contain up to 200 elements, including polyphenols and other antioxidants. It is a powerful antibacterial and has been shown to inhibit H. pylori growth. If the level of blood sugar is normal, honey can be use as sweetener without restriction.

Garlic

It has been proven that garlic extract inhibits H.pylori growth in lab, animal and human trials. To be used with moderation, as it acts as a blood thinner.

Cranberry

Its main effect is in the urinary tract infections, preventing the bacteria to settle on the walls of the bladder. Cranberry might also fight H. pylori. However, someone should be attentive with the quantity. The excessive consumption of cranberry might cause stomach discomfort. And also the commercial cranberry juices should be avoided, as they are sweetened with sugar and/or high fructose corn syrup, which can also cause stomach upset and add empty calories.

Fruits, vegetables and whole grains

It is important to have a vitamin-rich diet to prevent stomach ulcer. The aliments containing polyphenols – an antioxidant – prevent and also help ulcer healing.

Polyphenol-rich foods and seasonings include:

1. dried rosemary

2. Mexican oregano

3. dark chocolate

4. blueberries

5. black olives

Vitamin E

Doctors at the Kiev Medical Institute reported that 300 mg of vitamin E daily effectively treated peptic ulcers of 28 patients. Ulcers were relieved in four to six days in the vitamin E group, while it took seven to ten days in those given conventional medication. Patients taking vitamin E also had increased protein repair in their intestinal linings and gained from 1.5 to 3 kg during the study, while the controls did not gain any weight.

Cabbage

Decades before antibiotics, cabbage juice was successfully used to prevent or heal peptic and duodenal ulcers. In one study, it was shown that cabbage juice alone had a cure rate of over 92% in the treatment of these ulcers. This compared to about a 32 % cure rate in those using a placebo or other treatment. Cabbage is also a reliable source of vitamin C, which has been found to be lower in the gastric juice of ulcer patients.

Capsaicin

Hot chili peppers do not cause gastric ulcer. In fact, their consumption prevents ulcer development, because they trigger mechanisms that protect the lining of the stomach. Studies in Hungary found that consumption of capsaicin (the chemically active component in most peppers) actually decreased the acid output of the stomach, while at the same time increased protective secretions. In simple terms, peppers act as an antacid.

Bananas

These fruits contain an antibacterial substance that may inhibit the growth of ulcer-causing H. pylori. Studies show that animals fed bananas have a thicker stomach wall and greater mucus production in the stomach, which helps build a better barrier between digestive acids and the lining of the stomach.

To keep in mind

…do not hesitate to see your doctor for a proper diagnosis. Stomach ulcer symptoms should be taken seriously

… Are you sure you have a stomach ulcer? This is an important question because stomach ulcer symptoms can easily be confused with the symptoms of other gastrointestinal tract disorders

… H. pylori is becoming increasingly resistant to antibiotic treatments

… Approximately 65% of patients infected with H. pylori are simultaneously infected with Candida Albicans

… Many 'old school' doctors still hold on to the outdated 'No Acid, No Ulcer' mentality, and insist on treating the symptoms of Acid Reflux (GERD) only.

…Up to 90% of all types of stomach ulcers are caused by infections of Helicobacter Pylori, and not by spicy foods or by stress

… Helicobacter Pylori can easily be transmitted from person to person by kissing, and also through sexual contact

… In poorer countries, 50% of the population is infected with H. pylori in childhood, and up to 90% of adult populations are also infected

… The World Health Organization reported that H. pylori is present in 50% of all new gastric cancer cases

… Approximately 1 in every 8 people will develop duodenal ulcers or stomach ulcers in their lifetime.

…Stomach Ulcers affect more than 5 million people each year in the USA alone.

…Every year over 300,000 people round the world have ulcer related surgery because of persistent symptoms or complications.

…Each year nearly 6,000 people die of ulcer-related complications in the USA alone.

...Another major cause of ulcers is the prolonged use of aspirin and other painkillers, commonly known as NSAID's
...Nearly 3 in every 4 gastric ulcers are caused by H. pylori
...30% of people aged between 30 - 40 years are infected with H. pylori, as are 40% of people aged between 40 - 50 years being infected, and 50% of people aged between 50 - 60 years being infected, and so on
...People of any age can suffer from ulcers
...Women are just as prone to stomach ulcers as men are
...Peptic ulcers will affect nearly 1 in 10 of all adults in Western countries.
...About 1 in every 20 gastric ulcers leads to stomach cancer
...Duodenal ulcers may occur in adults of any age
...Gastric ulcers affect mainly adults older than 40 years
...The older you get, the more prone you will become to H. pylori infection

Questions and answers

How was the stomach ulcer treatment affected since the discovery of Helicobacter pylori as the main cause of it?
In the western world, this bacterium can be easily treated and has very rapidly disappeared. However, it remained a big issue in other parts of the world. The infection rate is of 70% in China and of 80% in India. In Eastern Europe is rated at 90%. The people infected with H. pylori are extremely susceptible of having in their lifetime stomach ulcers. Further, if not treated, the ulcer advances into gastric cancer. Gastric cancer is the second most usual cause of cancer death worldwide.
What is the most used treatment for stomach ulcer?

Most of the doctors use a triple therapy. It comprises 7-14 days of at least two types of antibiotics, together with a proton-pump inhibitor. The quadruple therapy consists of three types of antibiotics and a proton-pump inhibitor. Since the discovery of H.pylori and its treatment, it has remained the only infection that can be cured with antibiotics fully. Any other infections within the gastrointestinal system cannot completely be healed.

Do patients develop resistance to antibiotics?

Yes, they do. The *side effect* of using antibiotics for treating any other infection is that the patients develop a resistance to them. Even if it can be cured with the existent antibiotics, the infection with H. pylori does not benefit of an antibiotic especially created for it. Recent studies show that the failing rate of antibiotics treatment is of 1 in 5. In other words, from five patients with stomach ulcer that are under antibiotics, one is not responding.

Is there any solution for the antibiotic resistance?

One answer would be to discover other therapies or new antibiotics. Another solution is to assure treatment in two phases – sequential treatment. In the first phase, the patient uses an antibiotic with an acid inhibitor. The body becomes weaker and in the second phase, the antibiotics are more effective against the bacterium.

Is there any undergoing research for new antibiotics?

Yes, there are some companies working especially on developing antibiotics for H. pylori. The purpose of these is to be able to get in the gastric mucous layer, where the bacterium lives.

What is important for patients to know?

It is very important for a patient to know the efficiency of a treatment depends on its completion. And also, if the treatment is stopped halfway, it increases the risk of becoming resistant to antibiotics. Moreover, everyone should discuss with their health provider the side effects. Sometimes, if the patients are not aware, they can become scared of side effects and stop the treatment.

When should a person call the doctor?

A possible patient should see a doctor especially if the symptoms do not improve or reappear despite the treatment. Also, the doctor should be noticed if the symptoms get worse or if new symptoms appear.

What type of doctor should someone see, if presents any of the symptoms of stomach ulcer?

In cases of emergency, the person just has to call the hospital emergency number from the area they live in.

In other cases, some different types of health providers can be contacted: family medicine physicians, an internist, a general practitioner, a nurse practitioner, a physician assistant, or a pediatrician (for children and teenagers).

A family medicine physician is a medical doctor specialized in the total health care of the individual and the family. They have the expertise and the knowledge to diagnose and treat a wide range of health conditions and health problems, for males and females of all ages. Sometimes they can further specialize in some other area of medicine.

An internist is a medical doctor whose specialty is especially within the care of adults' area. They offer medical services such as regular checkups but can also prescribe treatment for a series of illness. Internists specialize in areas like: adolescent medicine, allergy, or immunology, cardiology (diseases and conditions of the heart and blood vessels), endocrinology (diseases of the endocrine glands, which regulate hormones), gastroenterology (diseases of the digestive system), geriatric medicine (conditions and diseases in older adults), hematology (diseases of the blood and blood system), infectious disease (complex infections), nephrology (diseases of the kidney and urinary system), oncology (cancer), pulmonology (lung diseases such as asthma, emphysema, and pneumonia), and rheumatology (immune system diseases and diseases of the joints).

A general practitioner is the one who has the knowledge and experience to diagnose and treat most of the health conditions or diseases, and they do not specialize in any specific domain of medicine. Usually, they provide basic medical services.

Nurse practitioners have high medical education and clinical training. They are able to do physical exams, diagnose and treat health issues, give medical information, order tests and prescribe medication. They can also specialize in different areas, such as care of children, of older adults, people of all ages, or persons with mental health problems.

The physician assistant is the one professional who practices medicine only under a doctor's supervision. Normally they have the abilities to take routine exams, to order lab work, prescribe medication and offer medical information.

If none of the medical specialists mentioned above cannot exactly diagnose a stomach ulcer, they might recommend the patient to see a gastroenterologist. They are the medical doctors specialized in diagnosis and treatment of diseases of the digestive system. Gastroenterologists can take specialized tests, such as endoscopy. In some situations they might coordinate their patient care with surgeons. Gastroenterologists may further specialize in treating people in certain age groups, such as pediatric gastroenterologists, who only treat children.

What should the patient discuss with the health provider?
Every patient has the right to plan their treatment. Also, they should know all the treatment options, discussed in detail with the medical doctors. The patient has the right to refuse treatment. However, no information available in this text or in any other sources should replace the specialized diagnosis and treatment.

www.ingramcontent.com/pod-product-compliance
Lightning Source LLC
Chambersburg PA
CBHW072029190526
45166CB00015B/1666